Back to Basics: Finding Wholehearted Ways to Wellness

by

Jennifer Manlowe, PhD, MDiv

Life Design Publishing

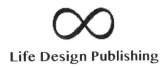
Life Design Publishing

First published in 2017 by **Life Design Publishing** Morristown, NJ
U.S.A.

Copyright © 2017 by Jennifer Manlowe.

ISBN-13:978-1542881050 - ISBN-10:1542881056

All rights reserved. This book, or parts thereof, may not be reproduced in any form without permission. For more information, contact Dr. Jennifer Manlowe at EmboldenU.com.

I dedicate this book to my mother, Susan Karr Kuebler

Back to Basics: Finding Wholehearted Ways to Wellness

In *Back to Basics,* psychology and religion scholar Jennifer Manlowe uses the term *wholehearted health* to mean *to cultivate wellbeing with the whole heart totally engaged.* She explores topics that include exercise, stress management, nutrition, social ties, community, environment and more.

Through the pages that follow, she inspires us to consider using specific exercises and questions as well as the latest findings in alternative healthcare. Exercises can be tailored to each reader's specific needs.

If put into action, *Back to Basics* will also help readers set goals and make lasting adjustments that complement the work they do with Dr. Manlowe as she helps clients balance life, work and wellness.

Whether you are looking to jump start your wellness program, prevent a long list of diseases through healthy lifestyle changes, or are looking for a healthy option to help transform a particular health challenge, *Back to Basics* will be a great choice for you!

~ Mishabae Mahoney, author and nutrition therapist, *Deeper Balance*

CONTENTS

What are the Basics of Wholehearted Wellness?

Finding Wholeheartedness

Understanding Ourselves

Understanding Our Environment

Physical Health

Emotional Health

Eating and Thinking Healthily

Regular Exercise

Can You Give Yourself a Break?

Sleep Habits

Getting Grounded

Sharing Ourselves with Others

Empathizing with Others

Setting Boundaries

Making and Keeping Friends

Maintaining Healthy Ties with Family

Becoming Curious about our Unfamiliar Neighbors (Near and Far)

Practicing Care for Our Surroundings (Wherever We Are)

Do Smartphones Make Us Dumb?

Build Courage

Joy is Not the Absence of Pain

Cultivating A Framework for Living

In times of life crisis, whether wildfires or smoldering stress, the first thing I do is go back to basics... am I eating right, am I getting enough sleep, am I getting some physical and mental exercise every day? ~ Edward Albert

If you give your life as a wholehearted response to love, then love will wholeheartedly respond to you. ~ Marianne Williamson

What Are the Basics of Wholehearted Wellness?

A goal I have for *Back to Basics: Finding Wholehearted Ways to Wellness* is to be inclusive of those eager to achieve health and wellness goals, no matter their starting point. This book grew up out of a wellness conversation begun with my own holistic health professional in the late 1990s. It was originally designed as an illness-prevention program to influence healthy lifestyle changes through adjusting life-long habits. After teaching philosophy, psychology and wisdom traditions and having more experiences with my own health and wellness challenges, I began to define wellness as something one pursues in a whole way vs. a holistic way (i.e., alternative medicine alone).

My focus here is the belief that we do not create our sense of wellness out of nowhere, rather we *return* to an innate sense wellness within each of us. Our foundation for living — "the basics" — can include the following habits and have found my own life (and my clients' lives) grow in health and wellness by practicing simple fundamentals, the same ones I lay before you in what's to follow.

Finding Wholeheartedness

Finding

Verb/Gerund

1. discovering, locating, uncovering or detecting (something or someone) with or without planning or trying to.

Wholeheartedness

Adjective

2. showing or characterized by complete enthusiasm, sincerity and commitment.

Enthusiasm comes from the ancient Greek word *En* "in" and *Theos* "spirit". To be enthusiastic means then "to have an indwelling of spirit" or in that ancient time period, to be "possessed by a [Greek] god's essence." One sees this enthusiastic spirit often in newlyweds, newly pregnant women, giddy children and anyone who has just fallen in love. Wouldn't it be great to feel this way all the time? Actually, we would be overrun with stress hormones (adrenaline and cortisol) and it wouldn't be *that* great for us!

In *Back to Basics*, I use the term *wholehearted health* to mean "an enthusiastic commitment to cultivating wellbeing." If you have not found this feeling yet, you might. If you are willing to experiment with at least one of these ways of finding wellness, you most certainly will. From my experience working with students and life-balance coaching clients, I have come to believe that wellness happens by engaging in body, mind and spirit activities.

When we make these habits priorities and effectively set boundaries to focus on them, we experience tangible shifts. Our overall health and satisfaction in both personal and relational endeavors bloom quite naturally. We're more able to focus and handle tension during stressful times. When we are out of balance we are able to make the necessary adjustments to restore our fundamental wellness.

The power that made the body, heals the body. ~ B.J. Palmer

Healing is the rediscovery of who we are and who we have always been.
~ Joan Borysenko

What we call "Alternative" medicine is generally defined as any of a range of medical therapies such as herbalism, homeopathy, and acupuncture, that are not regarded as orthodox by the medical profession.

"Holistic" medicine is a term used to describe therapies that attempt to treat the patient as a whole person. That is, instead of treating an illness, as in orthodox allopathy, holistic medicine looks at an individual's overall physical, mental, spiritual, and emotional wellbeing before recommending treatment.

"Orthodox"(from Greek ὀρθοδοξία, *orthodoxia*) is translated as "right opinion". Orthodox medicine is a system of medicine in which medical doctors, nurses and other healthcare professionals deliver treatment for diseases and their symptoms to the patients through the use of pharmaceuticals or surgery. Orthodox medicine is also known as "Western" medicine.

More and more health practitioners are beginning to see what they do as "whole health care". Such practitioners, as a rule, have the premise that you have an inborn intelligence that is programmed for self-healing, self-regulating, and the full expression of health. Even the staunchest Western-educated student of medicine works to hold off on looking for what's wrong, instantly diagnosing and prescribing drugs and waiting until all alternatives to surgery are exhausted before recommending that approach to chronic illness.

I am not one who was born with the possession of knowledge; I am one who is fond of antiquity and earnest in seeking it there. ~ Confucius

Confucius, the Chinese philosopher, born 551 B.C.E., put forward no claim to originality in all his writings. He spoke of himself as a compiler not a composer, a transmitter and not an inventor, believing in and loving the wise ones that came before him. This book, like his *Analects* — "book of sayings" — is merely bringing together what more of us are finding in a daily way, if we live like we matter, we will treat ourselves and others that way as well.

I find, unless you've abused your body so thoroughly as to cause organ shutdown, the body knows what feels healthy and what feels toxic. It is we who have failed to attune to its messages. We have to question our current contexts and ask, does this choice support or hinder my health? Does what I do hurt or help those I love, strangers, or the planet?

But first things first on the path to *returning* to wellness; we need to understand ourselves.

The body is wise, the confusion is from the mind. ~ Aniekee Tochukwu Ezekiel

I do not want the peace that passeth understanding. I want the understanding which bringeth peace. ~ Helen Keller

Understanding Ourselves

At one time or another we have all asked ourselves, "Why is this happening to me?" or "Why do I keep having the same problems?" or "Why am I hurting?" These difficult but important questions nudge us closer to a better understanding of ourselves and others. If our queries go unanswered, we become stuck in a cycle, continually repeating the past and forever on the defensive. Having some influence on our lives *requires* that we reflect on our lives.

When Thales of Miletus, one of the sages of ancient Greece, was asked, "What is difficult?" he is said to have replied, "To know yourself." Though the importance of self-knowledge — self-awareness — cannot be understated, it remains the most difficult task any of us face. But until you know yourself, strengths and weaknesses, you cannot succeed in any but the most superficial sense of the word.

Today we know that self-awareness is the ability to think about yourself and your relationship with the world around you. In his book *Emotional Intelligence,* behavioral psychologist Daniel Goleman describes self-awareness as "an ongoing attention to one's internal states." It is the ability to name and see how your emotions and perceptions are influencing your thinking and behavior. This is important because, all things being equal, more people lose relationships and employment by behavioral issues than by anything else. Our behavior is a reflection of our thoughts and as such can be changed for the good of all our relationships.

Clinical professor of psychiatry Daniel J. Siegel refers to it as <u>mindsight</u>. "Mindsight" describes our human capacity to perceive the mind of the self and others. He writes,

> It is a powerful lens through which we can understand our inner lives with more clarity, integrate the brain, and enhance our relationships with others. *Mindsight* is a kind of focused attention that allows us to see the internal workings of our own minds. It helps us get ourselves off of the autopilot of ingrained behaviors and habitual responses. It lets us "name and tame" the emotions we are experiencing, rather than being overwhelmed by them.

Careful reflection is no simple task and often goes underdeveloped because we tend to resist facing our vulnerabilities. Our vision of our inner world does not come as naturally to us as our ability to perceive the outside world. Yet to neglect our inner-life is to run on empty; even to hurt others (and ourselves) without consciously meaning to do so. The trick is to become conscious of our inner dialogue.

Mindsight or "careful reflection" nevertheless is a learnable skill that with some direction, time and effort can improve. It is not an all-or-nothing proposition but a continuum — an ongoing process that we engage in throughout life. The choice is ours as to how far we are willing to go to change the way we think and interact.

Unfortunately, most of us prefer what I call consumption-distraction — to consume something/anything as a way to avoid our inner challenges. We think, "I've done enough reflection and don't want to be a navel gazer." We take the easy way out and quit too soon. We find our habitual ways of thinking often work to maintain our personal comfort and, as such, we get in the way of our own growth and happiness. If we do a shallow job in our self-interrogation of thoughts, feelings and behaviors, we will get shallow results and unsatisfying relationships.

The good news, we need not keep the blinders on. With the help of *Back to Basics*, we can learn to welcome what scares us and change for the better.

Questions for Reflection

- When did you first hear, "That behavior is healthy or unhealthy?"
- Who taught you what is healthy?
- Where do you turn to today to learn what is healthy?
- What are differences between health and wellness as conceived by western medical doctors and alternative health providers?
- Identify where you are right now and where you would like to be in a year from now. Write a sentences about what's in the way of your progress.
- Why do we resist change? Why do we start off well and then lose steam?

The earth will not continue to offer its harvest, except with faithful stewardship. We cannot say we love the land and then take steps to destroy it for use by future generations. ~ Pope John Paul II

An understanding of the natural world and what's in it is a source of not only a great curiosity but great fulfillment. ~ David Attenborough

Understanding Our Environment

Believe it or not, where we live has a lot to do with how we perceive health and wellbeing. Whether we are born in a small town, a big city, a small village, an island or a farm, we will observe that people in our locale have a fairly similar idea of what is or is not healthy.

Aging and our approach to it is influenced by our social and cultural environment as well. Some cultures believe the elderly hold the most knowledge and should be looked to as experts in how to live well; they are held with great esteem as the ones that show us how to cultivate what makes a worthwhile life. They often pass on ancient myths and tell sacred stories that support change for every stage of the cycle of life.

In other cultures, like in the US, we look to popular heroes and heroines, psychologists, and medical experts (often online!), and, at times, we even look to Hollywood movie stars to tell us how to eat, exercise, think and behave in order to be happy. Oftentimes the focus on "health" is one dedicated to creating and maintaining a youthful appearance. Such an impossible pursuit is a solitary pursuit. We forget that our cultural surroundings and backward promises affect our sense of wellness in profound ways.

Understanding our environment includes considering not only social stressors but environmental ones as well. Consider the physical effects of noise, natural disasters, pollution, time pressures and negative news. Everyday life is also full of little irritations that accumulate overtime. If we use an alarm clock to wake up, the loud noise from the alarm is an environmental stressor. Extreme temperatures are also environmental stressors and can lead to discomfort. Other common environmental stressors include:

- LED lighting from our multiple technological devices
- Fluorescent lighting overhead in the workplace
- Crowding
- Sexism, homophobia, racism or religious intolerance in general
- Chemicals in cleaning and hygiene products we use everyday
- Air quality in traffic and caused by automobiles
- Prolonged exposure to dark surroundings
- Social tensions among groups (whether in our midst or in the world at large)
- Isolation and relating to others online vs. in person
- Violence or aggression in the home
- War, global warming and other human-made disasters

Recent research has linked extreme temperatures, crowding, and noise with increased levels of social aggression. Studies have also shown that crime rates are higher during the hottest days of summer. Exposure to natural light and fresh air can improve our mood and decrease fatigue, while prolonged exposure to darkness and stuffy indoor air can interfere with sleep patterns and lead to symptoms of depression.

Early in the 21st century, the World Health Organization (WHO) has acknowledged environmental pollution as tan underlying cause in nearly 80% of all chronic degenerative diseases. Toxic chemicals and metals have the potential to negatively influence every biological function occurring within our bodies.

Wellness, then, is an environmental issue. Knowing that we are influenced by our surroundings is the beginning of awareness of our environment and awareness is the beginning of choosing what restores us to our fundamental health and wellness.

Questions for Reflection

- Explain how your social and physical environments influence your health.
- What are differences between cultures as to "what is healthy"?
- How did your known ancestors conceive of "the good life" and "the basics" regarding health and wellness? If you don'y know, ask your older relatives.
- What did your parents practice as health and wellness basics? How are your current practices different?
- What elements of your environment place stress on you and those you care about?

Doctors of the future will give no medicine but will interest their patients in the care of the human frame, in diet and in the cause and prevention of disease. ~ Thomas Edison

A person too busy to take care of their health is like a mechanic too busy to take care of their tools. ~ Spanish Proverb

Physical Health

Physical wellness is something most of us aspire to; very few of us (over 40) are without complaint in terms of our mobility and sense of balance. When we are physically healthy, we usually feel happy in spirit and in our bodies. How do we measure physical health?

In ancient times, the gauge of wellness was a sense of mind-body balance. Even in the 21st-century, the Centers for Disease Control and Prevention (CDCP) write, "Health is a state of complete physical, mental, and social well-being, and not merely the absence of disease or infirmity."

When working at Brown University's School of Medicine, I was trained to conduct health research by the CDC. They had me use a questionnaire entitled Healthy Days Measures. Some of these questions include the following:

- Would you say that in general your health is excellent, very good, good, fair or poor?

- Now thinking about your physical health, which includes physical illness and injury, how many days during the past 30 days was your physical health not good?

- Now thinking about your mental health, which includes stress, depression, and problems with emotions, how many days during the past 30 days was your mental health not good?

- During the past 30 days, approximately how many days did poor physical or mental health keep you from doing your usual activities, such as self-care, work, or recreation?

One of the ways we think about our health is when it is missing. For instance, when we feel physical stress, we often have physical symptoms arise. Physical stress can be born of, or lead to, poor nutrition, poor sleep, and physical injury.

More of us are learning about how hormones affect our experience of wellness. Our bodies release adrenaline when we are stressed to help us have quick energy to cope. Whether the stress is physical or emotional, the effects of adrenaline in the body (especially for long periods) can be exhausting. Given all this, it is easy to see how stress causes excessive wear and tear that leaves us physically spent. Such burnout leads us to reach for artificial mood elevators, substances like fast foods, sugar, alcohol or drugs to relax. Almost all of us use caffeine to get a boost to keep going. By ingesting these chemicals, we've just doubled the amount of manageable stress.

For example, when we're in a panic over something, we become saturated with the stress hormones of adrenaline, cortisol and norepinephrine. This saturation results in a "shut down" response; a pattern that creates not only sleep deprivation and exhaustion but a sluggish metabolism. Experts agree, when we are not balanced energetically, we are more likely to shovel in quick energy, chemically-manufactured, and high-sugar foods. And as a result, we're nutritionally depleted and therefore more likely to crash in front of our favorite Netflix series to watch one show after the other until we pass out.

Shaking things up...

The human body is a complex system of bones, joints, muscles, and nerves designed to work together to accomplish one thing: motion. Even the ancient founders of the Olympic games, (in honor of the god Zeus), 2700 + years ago held the slogan "motion is life."

As a matter of fact, research has shown that motion is so critical to our health that a lack of motion has a detrimental effect on everything from digestion to our emotional state, immune function, our ability to concentrate, how well we sleep and even to how long we live. If our lifestyle does not include enough motion, our body becomes sluggish, achey and will no longer function efficiently.

According to a chiropractor named Dr. Richard Andreasen, there are three ways we know we are unhealthy: "First, you will not be as physically healthy and will suffer from a wide variety of physical ailments, ranging from headaches to high blood pressure. Second, you will not be as productive in your life because of reduced energy levels and the lack of ability to mentally focus. Third, because you have less energy, your activity level will tend to drop off even further over time, creating a downward spiral of reduced energy and less activity until you get to a point where even the demands of a sedentary job leave you physically exhausted at the end of the day."

Chiropractors also believe that the human body craves alignment and claim when properly aligned, our bones, not simply our muscles, support our weight, reducing effort and strain. The big payoff with proper posture is that we feel healthier, have more energy, and move gracefully. So while the word "posture" may conjure up images of book-balancing charm-school girls, it is not just about standing up straight. It is about being aware of and connected to every part of ourselves.

Maintaining mobility is critical in order to feeling good in our bodies, minds and spirits. Maintaining good mobility is not difficult for most of us, but it does not happen on its own. In developing good posture, it is necessary that we perform specific exercises and stretches to keep muscles, ligaments, and tendons flexible and healthy. In addition, it is necessary that all of the joints in our body are kept moving correctly as well. No need to buy expensive athletic equipment to stay flexible, this can be achieved to a great degree through stretching.

Questions for Reflection

- How do I take care of myself physically?
- How do I know when I'm out of balance physically?
- What small action am I willing to take to improve my physical range of motion?
- What are two stretches I love to do and two that I haven't yet tried?
- Am I willing to look up on WebMD.com or YouTube.com the best stretches for someone with my kind of body aches and pain? No need to do them, but they're there for you should you need an example.
- How will I celebrate progress in physical self-care?

Emotions are not problems to be solved. They are signals to be interpreted.
~ Vironika Tugaleva

I don't think that bravery is about skin. Bravery is about a willingness to show emotional need. ~ Richard Gere

Emotional Health

Emotional Health refers here to our overall psychological well-being. It includes the way we feel about ourselves, the quality of our relationships, our ability to manage feelings and deal with difficulties, and how much meaning and joy we derive from life. It isn't just the absence of mental health problems such as depression or anxiety. Rather, it's the presence of positive characteristics, such as being able to cope with life's challenges, handle stress, build strong relationships, and recover from setbacks that arise with even the most average of challenges.

Emotional health encompasses our reactions, in thought and emotion, to various stressors. Receiving criticism, for example, is devastating to some, while others seem unaffected. How do you know if what you're feeling is too much for the occasion? Who decides? Maybe you're just having a bad day or perhaps a rough few weeks. Are you just feeling down, a little anxious, irritable or are you feeling one breath away from the "last straw"?

Feeling blue, you may be surprised to learn, is quite common; most doctors and philosophers say it is part of the human condition. Charles Goodstein, MD, clinical professor of psychiatry at NYU Medical Center says, "The presence of anxiety, of a depressive mood or of a conflict within the mind, does not stamp any individual as having a psychological problem because, as a matter of fact, these qualities are indigenous to the species."

But, if living on the "last straw" has more or less become your way of life, experts say there is something on your mind that is crying out for your attention. The key is to ask yourself, "How often do I feel this high level of distress?" and "How bad does it get and how long does that level of stress last?" Such questions can help determine the seriousness of your situation.

When we feel emotionally healthy, just like when we feel physically healthy, we are probably having an overall sense of flexibility, resilience and balance. Cultivating emotional health is possible and even vital to a wholehearted sense of wellbeing. It doesn't have to be complicated.

In my wellness practice, I teach several forms of unplugging from unnatural stimulants in life. This does not mean no caffeine ever, rather it means noticing the effects of our over-stimulating environment and working to cut out 10-to-50% of those stressors.

I find it is easier to pick up good habits than to try to STOP COLD the old ones. Arriving just 10 minutes early to any appointment can give us time in the car (lobby) to gather ourselves, think about the day ahead, or even plan what healthy activity we will do to reward ourselves.

Instead of meeting a friend for coffee or a movie (sedentary and often involves food), meet them for a walk and a hearty visit. It meets our needs for social connection, raises our energy — even our metabolism — and relaxes us at the same time. Remember the wisdom of Socrates, "The unexamined life is not a life worth living." If we never pause to notice how we feel or what we are experiencing in the present, we may miss our body's signals for attention. And certainly, we will miss what is all around us, thus overlook the whole point of living fully.

If you have made consistent efforts to improve your mental and emotional health and still don't feel good, then it's time to seek help. Input from a knowledgeable, caring professional can often motivate us to do things for ourselves that we feel unable to do on our own. There are many resources to be accessed through your local Suicide Prevention Hotline. Here's how to find support in your area: 1-800-273-8255 — there's even an online format to talk to someone now (24/7).

Questions for Reflection

- How do you know when you are off balance emotionally?
- When you are feeling great inside, what seems to support or create that sensation?
- When you feel sad, mad, unsociable, or afraid how do you share these experiences vs. get bottled up and uncomfortable?
- What do you do when you are worried about your own or someone else's emotional wellness?

Our body is a machine for living. It is organized for that; it is its nature. Let life go on in it unhindered and let it defend itself, it will do more than if you paralyze it by encumbering it with remedies. ~ Leo Tolstoy

You don't get ulcers from what you eat. You get them from what's eating you.
~ Vicki Baum

Eating and Thinking Healthily

As I have said in the first chapter, "eating healthily" is often articulated differently depending on where you live. Although people do choose what to eat and drink, they can only choose from among foods and beverages that are available to them. If the food all around us is chemically altered, contaminated or highly processed, we won't have the best chance of eating a healthy diet.

Having healthy food choices is an important part of a healthy lifestyle. So many of us never ask where our foods and beverages come from. The trip from farm to fork is like a food stream. Far upstream, the source is the food supply, all the foods that farmers produce. Then the foods go through processing. These foods flow downstream through many outlets before they end up on a person's fork.

As I've said before, our weight is also affected by how we relate to stress in our lives. If we ingest too many toxic foods (sugars, processed foods, fried foods) and not enough of the whole foods (fruits, vegetables, whole grains and protein), this can create stress to the gut by causing inflammation and possible damage to the lining of the intestines due to malnutrition. Though it is hard to believe, many obese people (especially children) are suffering from malnutrition due to living on non-nutritive foods including "diet foods" labeled fat free, low-calorie, gluten- or sugar-free.

I agree with many experts that healthy eating is primarily about food and nutritional diversity. Consumption of a wide variety of whole foods, especially vegetables, fruits, legumes, whole grains and nuts, is particularly important.

Most nutrition and obesity studies have found that the safest bet to reaching and maintaining a physically healthy body is to consume less and exercise more — not through starving, *juicing*, renouncing fat and carbs, or working out like a weekend warrior but by caring for yourself as a way of life. As scientist Michael Pollan says, "Eat food, not too much, mostly plants."

Probably the first two words are most important. "Eat food" means to eat *real food* — vegetables, fruits, whole grains, and, yes, fish and meat — and to avoid what Pollan calls "edible food-like substances," those manufactured "foods" you have to unwrap from their packages.

Another gauge of real food is to ask yourself, *Will this food rot within a week?* Or consider this question: *Could my great grandmother find this food in her home?* If the answer is "No," it is toxic no matter how many times the word "natural" is written on its packaging.

Many of us need to change other things too, like the ways we live, our attitude towards our bodies, the ways we move and how we pace ourselves in our daily lives. But, did you know that being kind to ourselves can promote and help you maintain balanced weight.

"Great thoughts speak only to the thoughtful mind, but great actions speak to all humankind." ~ Theodore Roosevelt

Noticing our thoughts and actions…

How we talk to ourselves has a great deal to do with how we see the world around us, how we see ourselves.

At my life-work coaching business, EmboldenU, I bring diverse methods to work *with* you to make sure your entire body, and your relationship to it, is healthy, not just visually thinner or stronger looking. If you're not connected to your body's experience, you'll never treat it right. No matter how much weight you lose on a magic bullet diet, science shows you'll gain it back plus more. If what you put *into* your body changes but what you think about it doesn't change, that physical shift won't last.

Pursuing well-rounded balance in body, mind and spirit may include seeking nutritional counseling but aligning your wellness actions with your thoughts requires practice. Perhaps guidance can get you started and eventually well on your way to support long-lasting change.

My clients often pursue this by evaluating their current lifestyle, and where they want to be. We also look at the gap between the two before we co-create an overall wellness plan that is suited to their particular needs, physical ability and preferences. By functioning as their ally and holding them accountable to a new framework, steady progress is inevitable.

Studies show that people implementing a multi-faceted health program usually see better and lasting results. Notice I did not say the word *faster*.

What many people do not know is that by receiving regular guidance regarding intentions for thoughts and action, healthful goals can be achieved. When pressure is taken off us by witnessing social messages and our own self-talk, we feel more freedom to choose what will make us REALLY feel better, more flexible and more able to exercise without self-judging commentary. Also, as I've said above, by having less stress hormones running through us, we won't need to saturate our body with a "shut down" response; a pattern that creates not only stress, sleep deprivation/exhaustion but a sluggish metabolism.

Questions for Reflection

- Where do the foods I eat come from?
- What kind of variety am I having in my diet?
- Who taught me how to have a "healthy diet"?

Those who think they have no time for exercise will sooner or later have to find time for illness. ~ Edward Stanley

The reason I exercise is for the quality of life I enjoy. ~ Kenneth H. Cooper

Regular Exercise

With the steep rise in chronic diseases today, many of us have turned to a quick fix drug (often prescribed by a physician) without realizing how powerful a clean diet and exercise can be at managing and preventing many of our most common ailments. While the American College of Sports Medicine and the World Health Organization (WHO) recommend a minimum of 150 minutes per week of moderate-to-vigorous exercise, less than half of Americans regularly exercise. These numbers are even lower among elderly who are often discouraged about exercise programs. Only about 30% of Americans in this study meet the 150-minute time recommendations and about 36% report having sedentary lifestyles.

Aristotle said, "We are what we repeatedly do." It is no surprise then that we have a lot of screen-addicted couch potatoes suffering from all kinds of body pain. How can a new exercise program help us achieve optimal health? If we're not athletic, why exercise? Here are four good reasons:

1. It boosts metabolism.
2. It slows down degenerative effects of aging.
3. It reduces risk of disease.
4. It makes us feel good.

Metabolism: An article entitled <u>How to Boost Your Metabolism with Exercise</u> claims, "Your metabolism includes all the things your body does to turn food into energy and keep you going. Some people have a faster <u>metabolism</u> than others."

> *God grant me the serenity*
> *To accept the things I cannot change;*
> *Courage to change the things I can;*
> *And wisdom to know the difference.*
> ~ Reinhold Niebuhr

Some things that affect whether your metabolism is speedy or sluggish include what you cannot change, like your genetic code. Focus instead on what you can change that does make a difference: regular exercise. Muscle cells need a lot of energy, which means they burn a lot of calories. In fact, they burn more calories than fat cells, even when you're not exercising. So the time you spend working out — especially strength training — reaps benefits long after you stop sweating.

Aging: Exercise becomes even more important as you get older. You naturally lose muscle mass with age, which slows down your metabolism. Working out can stop that slide and even reduce dementia risks, improve sleep, reduce stress and increase chances of never needing surgery. If surgery is ever needed, those who exercise regularly, even three days a week have been shown to bounce back much more quickly than their sedentary peers.

Disease: By exercising just 150 minutes per week, diabetes risks have been demonstrated to be reduced by 58%! Exercise is also effective at drastically reducing the risks for just about any chronic disease, including cancer, arthritis and heart disease. It effectively reduces inflammation and excess body fat, making it a powerful tool to improve your all around health and relieve any aches and pains on stressed-out/unused joints.

Feeling Good: Depression is rising among first-world people. If rates continue as they are, it will be the most prominent disease by 2020. A major cause of depression can be due to stress — overwork, underpay, financial fears, lack of sleep, unrealistic expectations, etc. But exercise has been shown to improve sleep, reduce stress and increase self-confidence. Studies consistently show that active individuals are less likely to have mental health problems. Exercise is not only great for staying in shape but is also a drug free way to elevate your mood.

Questions for Reflection

- When were you first exposed to someone else speaking about the importance of exercise?
- Which athlete(s) in history inspires you the most?
- When you feel down, what are the habits that precede it and/or relieve it?
- When your body feels sluggish, what's the first thing you do? How often do you let yourself move outdoors in ways that enliven you?
- What ways might you increase invigorating and enjoyable forms of outdoor activity?

You can do anything, but not everything. ~ David Allen

*Rest is not idleness, and to lie sometimes on the grass
under trees on a summer's day,
listening to the murmur of the water,
or watching the clouds float across the sky,
is by no means a waste of time.*
~ John Lubbock

Can You Give Yourself a Break?

Relaxing is never easy if you were raised in a "Type A" culture like the United States. Almost every country in the world works less than 40 hours a week. Japan and Germany are exceptions and, if you think about it, both of these "type A" countries have gone to war with us. What's the common denominator? Pushing ourselves to the breaking point as a daily habit. Perhaps going to war wasn't only about preserving freedom and democracy, perhaps it was also about the downside of the industrial revolution — its soul-crushing worker exhaustion, agitation, insecurity and fear.

How do we cope with these stressful demands? Today, so many people turn to prescribed (and even non-prescribed) medication or unhealthy habits to relax when they are stressed. [CDC Statistics](#) and other [Statistics](#) show.

- There were over 3.3 billion prescriptions filled in America in 2002 (12 times the US's population — that is 12 prescriptions for every man, woman, and child in the US that year).
- Paxil and Zoloft, two of the more popular anti-anxiety medications, ranked 7th and 8th in the top ten prescribed medications in the US (these two medications totaled almost $5 Billion in sales in 2002)
- 42% of young adults in America regularly use recreational drugs (National Institute on Drug Abuse).
- 48.7% of North Americans using at least one prescription drug in the past 30 days: 48.7% (2009-2012)
- 21.8% using three or more prescription drugs in the past 30 days: (2009-2012)
- 10.7% of persons using five or more prescription drugs in the past 30 days: (2009-2012)
- 43% take mood-altering, non-prescribed prescription drugs regularly.
- Alcohol is commonly used to cope with anxiety. In 1998, 50% of all traffic fatalities were alcohol-related (CBC Report).
- 25% to 40% of all patients in US hospitals are being treated for complications resulting from alcohol related problems (The Marin Institute).
- Alcohol-related car crashes are the number one killer of teens.
- Alcohol use is also associated with homicide, suicide, and drowning — the next three leading causes of death among youth (Center for Substance Abuse Prevention).

When it comes to changing habits of seeking relaxation, there is some good news. For instance, more of us are learning how to relax without altering our consciousness artificially. For instance:

- More of us are learning some form of soothing practice to calm our hearts and minds.
- According to the NIH, approximately 21 million adults (nearly double the number from 2002) and 1.7 million children practiced yoga.
- Nearly 20 million adults and 1.9 million children had chiropractic manipulation.
- Nearly 18 million adults and 927,000 children practiced meditation.
- Children whose parents use a complementary health approach are more likely to use one as well.
- Mindfulness Meditation has become mainstream in America and central to the mental health profession and is commonly used in the treatment of attention-deficit hyperactivity disorder, depression, anxiety, obsessive-compulsive disorder, personality disorders, substance abuse, post-heart attack rehabilitation and autism.
- More of us are simplifying our lives versus chasing bigger and better material wealth and the stress that comes with maintaining that demanding lifestyle.
- Lots of people are job sharing (20-hours-a-week each) or working a four-day week (if they can afford to do so).

More Americans of all ages are rolling out their yoga mats in an effort to improve their health. A large nationally-representative survey shows that the number of Americans using mind and body approaches to improve health and well-being remains high. Of note is a significant increase in the use of yoga since 2002. In addition, almost as many Americans practice meditation or receive chiropractic manipulation.

I've come to discover for myself what I've always heard as a student of both Eastern and Western philosophy that change is possible and the body's essential nature seeks balance and health. I believe with the right support, people who cannot seem to relax will be able to:

- Regain control of their health and life
- Live a balanced, happy, and fulfilling life
- Have happier and more fulfilling relationships
- Become the individual they always thought they could be
- Reconnect with life in a more rewarding and satisfying way
- Live an unrestricted lifestyle ready to tackle any challenge
- Express themselves like never before
- Live a more accepting life, appreciating uniqueness and imperfection
- Experience a more stable work environment
- Become free from drug use

Questions for Reflection

- How do you unwind after a challenging or busy day? List five ways you usually relax.
- Does anyone you know struggle with habits that disconnect them from being present with themselves and others?

- List ten new ways you could transform your own unhealthy "relaxation" habits.
- Are you willing to learn more about <u>mindfulness meditation</u> or yoga?

Sleep Habits

Your life is a reflection of how you sleep, and how you sleep is a reflection of your life. ~ Dr. Rafael Pelayo

Sleep is the best meditation. ~ Tenzin Gyatso, the 14th Dalai Lama

In 2010, the CDC research revealed one in six adults with a diagnosed sleep disorder. One in eight adults with trouble sleeping reported using sleep aids. They also found that 4% of US adults aged 20 and over used prescription sleep aids in the past month and the percentage of adults using a prescription sleep aid increased with age and education. More adult women (5.0%) used prescription sleep aids than adult men (3.1%).

Non-Hispanic white adults were more likely to use sleep aids (4.7%) than non-Hispanic black (2.5%) and Mexican-American (2.0%) adults. Prescription sleep aid use varied by sleep duration and was highest among adults who sleep less than five hours (6.0%) or sleep nine or more hours (5.3%).

When I had trouble sleeping during a very stressful time in my life after 9/11, my Western health practitioner recommended that I "take 1mg of Valium about 20 minutes before bed each night." He declared, "Many people with type A personality have hyperactive mental habits that are difficult to turn off naturally." While I didn't like the term "hyperactive," I did agree that "winding down" with acupuncture, biofeedback, meditation, yoga, etc.

never seemed to help. Like many Americans, I tried the pharmaceutical method for helping me get rest. Ten years later I found myself unable to fall asleep without this drug. If I traveled to a conference or on vacation and forgot this drug, I spent the night staring at the ceiling or tossing and turning. This was extremely disturbing AND inconvenient!

A few years ago, I met an acupuncturist who told me, "Valium is extremely addictive and it will be very hard to wean yourself off of." He worked with me over the course of six months to make smoother this very uncomfortable process. Now, I fall asleep easily on my own. Staying asleep is not as easy but today I use breathing meditation to relax and lull myself to sleep when I find myself wide awake at 2:00 AM.

In my own research I've learned there are multiple methods to share that foster a return to balance no matter what is happening within or outside of us. Relaxation techniques, meditation and contemplation, hypnosis and similar approaches can all have a strong mediating effect on stress that keeps us up at night.

We all know that stress will come. If you uncover your "hot buttons" or "triggers" and know who pushes them, you'll be able to treat the source rather than need to medicate the symptom of sleeplessness. What helps some of my clients is to take 10 minutes each night to organize things for the next day and to be reasonable in plans regarding what they can achieve in one day. This helps them proceed through the day in confidence and stay focused.

After decades of research, it is clear that the negative effects associated with stress are real. Although you may not always be able to avoid stressful situations, there are a number of things that you can do to reduce the effect that stress has on your body. The first is relaxation.

Just as each individual with show signs of stress differently, each individual needs to figure out their own path to relaxation. Below are four of the most common ways to relieve stress naturally:

Relaxed Breathing

Practice this basic four-by-four or **box technique** twice a day, every day, and whenever you feel tense. This is how it works:

* **Inhale.** With your mouth closed and your shoulders relaxed, inhale as slowly and deeply as you can to the slow count of four. As you do that, push your stomach out. Allow the air to fill your diaphragm.
* **Hold.** Keep the air in your lungs as you slowly count to four.
* **Exhale.** Release the air through your mouth as you pull your bellybutton gently in the direction of your spine and slowly count to four.
* **Hold.** Keep the air in your lungs as you slowly count to four.

Repeat the inhale-hold-exhale-hold cycle two to four times.

Progressive Muscle Relaxation

The goal of progressive muscle relaxation is to reduce the tension in your muscles. First, find a quiet place where you'll be free from interruption. Loosen tight clothing and remove your glasses or contacts if you'd like.

Tense each muscle group for at least five-seconds and then relax for at least 10 seconds. Repeat before moving to the next muscle group.

Upper part of your face. Lift your eyebrows toward the ceiling, feeling the tension in your forehead and scalp. Relax. Repeat.
Central part of your face. Squint your eyes tightly and wrinkle your nose and mouth, feeling the tension in the center of your face. Relax. Repeat.

Lower part of your face. Clench your teeth and pull back the corners of your mouth toward your ears. Show your teeth like a snarling dog. Relax. Repeat.

Neck. Gently touch your chin to your chest. Feel the pull in the back of your neck as it spreads into your head. Relax. Repeat.

Shoulders. Pull your shoulders up toward your ears, feeling the tension in your shoulders, head, neck and upper back. Relax. Repeat.

Upper arms. Pull your arms back and press your elbows in toward the sides of your body. Try not to tense your lower arms. Feel the tension in your arms, shoulders and into your back. Relax. Repeat.

Hands and lower arms. Make a tight fist and pull up your wrists. Feel the tension in your hands, knuckles and lower arms. Relax. Repeat.

Chest, shoulders and upper back. Pull your shoulders back as if you're trying to make your shoulder blades touch. Relax. Repeat.

Stomach. Pull your stomach in toward your spine, tightening your abdominal muscles. Relax. Repeat.

Upper legs. Squeeze your knees together and lift your legs up off the chair or from wherever you're relaxing. Feel the tension in your thighs. Relax. Repeat.

Lower legs. Raise your feet toward the ceiling while flexing them toward your body. Feel the tension in your calves. Relax. Repeat.

Feet. Turn your feet inward and curl your toes up and out. Relax. Repeat.

Perform this progressive muscle relaxation at least once or twice each day to get the maximum benefit. Each session should last about 10 minutes.

Exercise

Exercise is a good way to relieve pent-up energy and tension. It also helps us get in better shape, which makes us feel better overall. By getting physically active, we decrease our levels of anxiety and stress and elevate our moods. Numerous studies have shown that people who begin exercise programs, either at home or at work, demonstrate a marked improvement in their ability to concentrate, are able to sleep better, suffer from fewer illnesses, suffer from less pain and report a much higher quality of life than those who do not exercise. This is even true of people who had not begun an exercise program until they were in their 40s, 50s, 60s or even 70s. So if you want to feel better and improve your quality of life, get active!

Making Your Sleep Routine Your Own

Experts acknowledge that most people find it difficult to follow all these recommendations; however, they also stress that it isn't typically necessary to do so. They suggest that people identify the factors that are most disruptive to their own sleep and then focus on altering particular behaviors and patterns to overcome these factors.

Questions for Reflection

- When you have trouble sleeping, what seems to help you get back to it?
- If you looked back over the times in your life when you lost the most sleep, what seems to have motivated this reaction.

- What rituals are you willing to experiment with to aid you in sleeping well?
- What techniques would you add to the brief strategies I've laid out above?

Your vision will become clear only when you look into your own heart. Who looks outside, dreams. Who looks inside, awakes. ~ Carl Jung

In dwelling, live close to the ground. ~ Laozi

Getting Grounded

You're grounded! Why does this word grounded sound like a bad idea? Where did we get this negative association?

When we think of "being grounded" we think of being in trouble; with having restrictions placed on our movement or privileges. Some of us may recall days spent locked in our homes instead of with playing with friends on weekends or after school. In this case "being grounded" is considered a punishment for doing something wrong.

As adults, our other associations with the term "grounded" may have to do with travel and inconvenience. Think of an airplane flight you counted on to take you from one place to another. If it's grounded, it is being stopped or thwarted in some way.

In either scenario above, we're being kept from our preferences. Ironically, getting "un-busy" can feel like a form of punishment to those of us with *Type A* personalities. Stopping for us feels like we are being punished, or even punishing ourselves.

Once, Dr. Manlowe participated in a distressing seminar with other health professionals who were used to living a hectic life on and off hours. These professionals were missionaries dedicated to helping people prevent or heal from various illnesses.

The seminar leader asked the health providers to "not do" for twenty minutes a day. More than a few of the doctors claimed to have a rigorous meditation practice that they never missed. The leader said, "No, I'm not asking you to meditate. As a matter of fact, do not meditate. Rather, just stare out the window or go for a 20 minute stroll (not an aerobic walk or run). She had her pupils report back each day of the week and not one of these people could do this. They said, "I don't have time to waste." Or "I got too antsy not accomplishing anything; at least with meditation, I'm working toward a peaceful mind."

Imagine, the very people we see to show us how to become healthy cannot themselves muster the practices required to do so.

When we speak of "getting grounded" we're not asking you to do nothing. Rather, we mean learning habits that support us in getting off the treadmill and getting relaxed with ourselves. We're not talking about crashing after a long push to accomplish our "to do" list. We mean making time — vs. *finding time* — to pause and reflect on the need to "regroup."

It's like having a "huddle" with ourselves to ground ourselves in our intentions for a wholehearted life. It's a time to reflect, perhaps write in order to connect to our center. We both believe we benefit from time that neither plays hard or work hard, a time that is what some call gray. Where we get used to not accomplishing anything.

If we do anything, it's to re-member who we are and what matters to us right now. Some use the metaphor "tending to the garden" of our lives. When we do not make time for this, the ground dries up and dreams and relationships suffer, if not disappear altogether.

Questions for Reflection

- What happens when you stop doing anything? What feelings arise?
- When was the last time you drove in your car without listening to the radio or a favorite CD?
- What do you do, if anything, to calm your mind when you feel chaotic or that things are getting out of hand in terms of too busy.
- Who do you associate with someone who seems "grounded"? What does she or he prioritize to cultivate such a way of being?

Research shows that even brief autobiographical sharing exercises can have substantial impacts on psychological and physical health even months after.
~ Sherry Hamby

If we have no peace, it is because we have forgotten that we belong to each other. ~ Mother Teresa

Sharing Ourselves with Others

They say a problem shared is a problem halved. Now a team of psychologists in the USA has performed a series of studies that suggest sharing your good news multiplies its benefits for happiness and longer-term life satisfaction.

Dr. Christian Jarrett writes for *The British Psychological Society* and says, "Sharing is fundamental to the development of all human relationships and civilizations." We begin learning to share as soon as we are able to communicate. Often it begins with our parents teaching us the importance of sharing a toy with a friend or a sibling. In the mind of a toddler, this idea seems absurd at first. They think, "Why would I want to give up this awesome thing I'm playing with?" But even at that young age, they quickly realize the payoff. And what is it? It is the joy they feel when they see the happiness they have brought someone else.

Every tradition in the world comes down to one phrase, "Love your neighbor as yourself." Even Confucius said the same thing a little differently, "Do not do to your neighbors that which you would not want them to do to you." Not only does sharing bring us joy, it teaches us the importance of taking care of others. In many cultures, it is quite common to share your home with your elders.

It is important to know that sharing does not have to be a grand gesture to be appreciated. It can be as simple as sharing something you feel with someone, like a compliment. "You look great today," is one example. Those simple words can often make someone feel special and cared for, and in return, make the one who said this to them happy. Sharing is truly a win-win!

One of the best things you can share with others is your own happiness. Tell them what made you happy and why. Your story just might inspire a change in them. The next time something good happens to you, do not keep it to yourself. Why? My grandmother said it well: "Happiness held is the seed; happiness shared is the flower."

Questions for Reflection

- What were you taught about sharing your personal feelings with others?
- Who did you see as the most joyful relative?
- What kind of compliment lights you up?
- When have you done something nice for another without expecting anything in return? How did that make you feel?

Change begins with understanding and understanding begins by identifying oneself with another person: in a word, empathy. The arts enable us to put ourselves in the minds, eyes, ears and hearts of other human beings.
~ Richard Eyre

It is an absolute human certainty that no one can know his own beauty or perceive a sense of his own worth until it has been reflected back to him in the mirror of another loving, caring human being. ~ John Joseph Powell

Empathizing with Others

Most people think about empathy as feeling each other is pain but if you can <u>feel someone else's pleasure,</u> as our essay above states, you are a much happier person in general because it simply brings more joy into your life. Still, empathy must be cultivated in a culture fixated on getting more safety and security for ourselves or even for the ones we love.

Maia Szalavitz, author of *Born for Love: Why Empathy is Essential — and Endangered*, explains, "Empathy has two parts, a mental part and an emotional part."

- The mental part is the ability to put yourself in the mind of another, to see the world through someone else's eyes.
- The emotional part is caring about what the other person feels and experiences.

Sociopaths have the mental type of empathy, but not the emotional aspect; they can take other people's perspectives but they use this skill to manipulate and hurt them, not to help. People with autism often have problems with the mental type of empathy; they have difficulty with perspective-taking, but once they realize that other people have different thoughts and feelings, they can care very deeply about them and can sometimes even be overwhelmed by empathy.

In sum, empathy (the radical openness to the goodness of the other) opens the way to sympathy (when one accepts this openness). This enables us to care *about* the other and eventually care *for* the other.

Doing good for the other is just as easy, if not easier, than doing the good for ourselves. This bond not only breaks through the drive for a more-for-me approach to life, but also creates the condition for generous and even self-sacrificial love. This powerful drive forms the basis for another kind of desire, the desire to make a positive difference to someone or something beyond ourselves.

As the Dalai Lama says, "If you want to suffer, think only of yourself."

Questions for Reflection

- When you think about the suffering in the world, what makes you the saddest?
- How do you show care for others (including animals)?
- Would you say you're a good or bad listener? From your history, give an example of each.
- Are you willing to practice listening to another without interrupting or giving advice?

Good fences make good neighbors. ~ Robert Frost

"No" is a complete sentence. ~ Anne Lamott

Setting Boundaries

Boundaries aren't just a sign of a healthy relationship with ourselves and others; they're a sign of self-respect. When we never say no to our "to do" list, we're ruled by it. Stress follows and our sense of wholehearted wellness goes out the window. Learning to make time for ourselves requires self-respect, and it builds self-esteem as well. Letting ourselves be ruled by work or certain relationships will leave us feeling out of control. Overtime this can make us feel helpless and eventually hopeless, even depressed.

Many people who suffer from high blood pressure are shown to have a history of keeping their feelings and needs to themselves. The old cowboy or cowgirl image of John Wayne might have been their role model growing up. Now, most of us know there is nothing good about stuffing our feelings or pretending we don't have needs; those repressive habits could kill us.

But how do we exercise healthy boundaries with those we want to please, like our loved ones, our colleagues or employers? We find these techniques to be very helpful *and* healthful:

- If you're asked to do something you do not feel will improve yourself or your relationships, it's okay to say, "No thank you" or "No." As

Lamott says, "No is a complete sentence if you think about it." If you're not sure of your answer, it's okay to say, "I'm not sure about that; I'll get back to you by the end of the day tomorrow."

- Use "I" statements and feeling words to articulate preferences and needs. For example:

Working out before work helps me feel great, focused and more productive. I would love to come into work at 9:30 and leave at 5:30. Will that work for you?

OR

Spending an overnight with my gal pals once a month helps me feel giddy and relaxed. I feel refueled for my duties of managing our family business. What would help you decompress each month? I think we both deserve this kind of break from our regular routines.

OR

Kids, your mother and I have asked your favorite Aunt Mel to stay with you a few nights a month so we can have a special time alone together. It helps us grow and will be good for the entire family. How does that sound?

If we take the time to protect our time alone and with friends with healthy boundaries, everybody wins.

Questions for Reflection

- How does it feel to imagine making time for your health?
- Can you ask for what you want from your friends, family, colleagues, employers?
- Recall a time when someone asked something of you and seemed timid about it. How did that make you feel?
- Be willing to practice (role play) making a scary request with someone you feel safe in doing so.

True friendship is like sound health, the value of it is seldom known until it is lost. ~ C.C. Colton

The only way to have a friend is to be one. ~ Ralph Waldo Emerson

Making and Keeping Friends

Healthy relationships are a vital component of health and wellbeing. There is compelling evidence that strong relationships contribute to a long, healthy, and happy life. Conversely, the health risks from being alone or isolated in one's life are comparable to the risks associated with cigarette smoking, blood pressure, and obesity.

Research shows that healthy relationships can help you:

- **Live longer**. "People with social support have fewer cardiovascular problems and immune problems, and lower levels of cortisol — a stress hormone," says Tasha R. Howe, PhD, associate professor of psychology at Humboldt State University. One review of 148 studies found that people with strong social relationships are 50% less likely to die prematurely.

- **Deal with stress**. The support offered by a caring friend can provide a buffer against the effects of stress. In a study of over 100 people, researchers found that people who completed a stressful task experienced a faster recovery when they were reminded of people with whom they had strong relationships.

- **Be healthier**. According to research by psychologist Sheldon Cohen, college students who reported having strong relationships were half as likely to catch a common cold when exposed to the virus. "There may be broader effects as well," Cohen says. "Friends encourage you to take better care of yourself. And people with wider social networks are higher in self-esteem, and they feel they have more control over their lives."

- **Feel richer**. A survey by the National Bureau of Economic Research of 5,000 people found that doubling your group of friends has the same effect on your wellbeing as a 50% increase in income!

Remember, it's never too late to build new friendships or reconnect with old friends. Investing time in making friends and strengthening your friendships can pay off in better health and a brighter outlook for years to come. We are social animals and like most animals we travel in packs. It is in our DNA.

Questions for Reflection

- Where do I turn for social support?
- What have I learned about making and keeping friends?
- When have I felt most lonely?
- When have I felt the least healthy? Who was I hanging out with at the time?
- Who do I call my tribe? Who would I like in my tribe?

All human happiness revolves around love. Love is central to the bonds on which a family is built. ~ Margaret Way

If there's one thing I've learned over the eons, it's that you can't give up on your family, no matter how tempting they make it. ~ Rick Riordan

Maintaining Healthy Ties with Family

Research has proven time and again that dining together as a family promotes lifelong healthy eating habits. So many people who make the time, find that the benefits of this practice include improved communication, helping each member feel heard and seen and just a sense of overall fun. If you have a family of your own and dinner isn't already a part of your routine, aim for at least one meal a week together and build from there.

Family game night: In an age of seclusion via personal electronic devices, families tend to be a bit disconnected. As corny as this sounds, ask a friend what they do when they're not online. My grandmother suggests I think about the days before microtechnology. I learned that some families get back in sync by playing board games. Another family I know introduced games of strategy, brainteasers, charades or puzzles. It helps if you make no-tech nights a permanent "activity" on your calendar to ensure the whole family can leave room for it in their schedules.

Get active together: It doesn't matter if you're swinging at the park, canoeing across mountain lakes, or horseback riding across desert dunes —

getting active outside as a family is a great way to connect. Try a new sport or hike a new trail to keep your family interested and excited. If you're willing, get to know your neighbors or your kids' friends parents by playing team sports that fit each season.

No need to be politically conservative to have "family values". Find where you and your family members are "on the same page," ideologically, and focus on these values. If you don't know where your kids' or parents' principles stand, consider writing down your family's beliefs, goals, and aspirations. Allowing every family member to be involved in the process will encourage dialogue. Be sure to show the reasons behind each belief or goal and explain how remaining loyal to them will benefit the family as a whole.

If this applies to you, attend faith-based outings together: Faith has been a part of my life in varying degrees. Does your faith or philosophy resonate with your past? Is it new for you to think about it? Or has it been/become a focal part of your life. Becoming involved with a spiritual or civic community can support each member of a family. Service to others is a common theme in all traditions. Tithing is also important and even if you don't have a lot of dollars to share, offering a small portion of your income or some time helping others, you are adding to the goal of creating a better world.

All happy families are alike; each unhappy family is unhappy in its own way.
~ Leo Tolstoy

My own experience of family

I grew up in the Pacific Northwest the youngest of four in a Roman Catholic home. My Scottish mother was raised in Seattle in an agnostic home and converted to Catholicism in order to marry my Italian Catholic father, also raised in Seattle. In parochial school, we kids attended mass each morning of the week. As a family, we rarely missed Sunday mass but maintaining faith *within* the family was complicated for me. Remaining faithful proved impossible for my father who suffered from various addictions and mental health challenges. I grew up, then, in what many called a "broken home." I now see it as a "heartbroken" home.

Getting divorced as a Catholic in the 1960s meant being excommunicated from the church. This alienating act in my mind wounded all of us emotionally as well as spiritually. My father was gone by his own volition leaving my mother to raise four kids on her own, one of them with a serious developmental disability. Even though my dad was the only vow breaker, my very religious mother was forbidden to partake in "the communion meal" — she had to stay seated during the entire sacred ceremony. I felt shame watching her be *benched* for my father's sins. Seemed the expansive love of God preached from the pulpit was there for only some families.

Like many kids of a single parent, we pulled together and did whatever we could to stay strong and dignified as a family. Maintaining family ties was something we all tried to do, but there was a great deal of pain about the bonds that failed to mend. We kids had trouble believing that our dad was never coming back home. As a result of this tumult, I struggled to find hope.

My mother met a kind Episcopal man and married him. But, in the eyes of the church, their nuptials did not change her status as a woman held back from the communion meal. Before my mother would be allowed to again receive communion, she had to go before a Catholic tribunal of male judges/priests and, like Joan of Arc, defend her qualifications. For her new marriage to be deemed legitimate, her husband had to convert to Catholicism and she had to renounce ever having consummated her first marriage for an annulment — an act I understood as meaning all four of us children illegitimate. Somehow this patriarchal theater made sense to these adults and most especially to my mother, a Catholic convert. Later I learned that not all annulments require virginity on behalf of the female.

This patriarchal litigiousness baffled me and made me terribly angry. I was sure these judgmental rules were anti-female and contradictory to the inclusive message of Jesus, the one in whose name this church was founded. At age 10, I felt called to the priesthood to undo this damage and was determined to set it aright. In my teens, I discovered females were not allowed to be ordained. This only confirmed my concern that the Church of my family seemed threatened by female power. Why, then, would my mother want any part of it, I wondered?

With age, I learned to find hope by pursuing gender justice and learning from the most politically progressive Catholic mystics. A little later, in my 20s, I would attend Seminary and get my doctorate in the field of psychology of religion. I became one-pointed in my dedication to understanding how Christian faith can help or hurt families.

If religious dogma of any faith is patriarchal, it can ostracize women and stymie girls as it did my mother and myself. If doctrines of any sect promote communal engagement, inspire social and psychological growth, and support liberation for all, there is hope. As to gender justice, I came to see that only the ignorant and insecure refuse to admit when they are wrong. My job has not been to educate institutionally-religious people rather it's been to discover the values I believe and pursue them wholeheartedly. Looking to see where any religious tradition is just and loving, and fanning those flames, is my current practice.

Being a family member who prioritizes connection remains paramount to me and my family of origin. We continue to agree to resist letting our differences or the hardest parts of our past mar the present or sour the future. As a matter of course, we make time to be together regularly (for sports, movies, or potlucks). We sometimes travel together and never miss holidays or birthdays. While our particular constellation of family is different, our expression of spirituality and politics our own, there is one thing upon which we all agree, life without the bonds of family is untenable. There is no rift too great to be mended.

Whether one comes from an ordinary "happy family" *a la Tolstoy* or one like my own, family ties make a difference in our health and wellness. Recent social scientific research reveals the same.

At *The American Sociological Association* annual meeting in Seattle (2016), social scientist James Iveniuk found that elders without family ties of any kind had a greater risk of suffering a heart attack or stroke. He found "Family appears to be more important than friends because of what people expect from family." He reported, "We find it is common for people to think their family should be there to take care of them when in need, especially when ill or incapacitated in some way." Iveniuk explained. In contrast, "friends are more likely to move in and out of your network" and do so in many cases to take care of their own family responsibilities.

This is not to say that family is always better for you. Iveniuk believes, "There are lots of cases where family is burdensome, frustrating or even abusive, and you should not associate with them just because they are family."

For most people, most of the time, family are people with whom you are most likely to be close and more likely to be open about things like your health. Working to mend past pains or misunderstandings, if this applies to you, is worth doing. If for no other reason, our relations with family members make a significant difference in our joyful longevity.

Questions for Reflection

- On what occasions have I felt close to family?
- On what occasions have I felt estranged from family?
- Is there anyone in my family I need to talk to but resist doing so? Why?
- What small action can I take to have better relationships with my family? (This action may mean being more assertive or having better boundaries.)
- What would it take to engage with family members in ways that support all of us?
- Am I willing to speak up on behalf of maintaining family ties, especially with extended family members and in-laws, (if that applies)?

The compulsion to see what lies beyond the far ridge or that ocean — or this planet — is a defining part of human identity and success. ~ David Dobbs

For at least one moment, be fascinated by every human being. A thrilling mystery of life is walking right by you. Look closely. ~ Rabbi Noah Weinberg

Becoming Curious about our Unfamiliar Neighbors (Near and Far)

From the Daoist immortals to the Ancient Greeks, wise people have been asking, "Who is the wisest person?" And philosophers of every stripe answer, "The one who learns from every person."

Brian Glazer, author of [A Curious Mind: The Secret to a Bigger Life](#), claims even ordinary conversations can be a curiosity conversation if we try to learn something new from people we meet. It starts by getting curious. Glazer gives us a few practical tips on how to learn from every person.

1. **Learn from the unique challenges of every person.** To be human is to struggle. No matter how perfect a person's life appears on the outside, everyone is struggling with something. Maybe it is health. Maybe it is finances. Maybe it is a difficult relationship. Understanding others' battles can help us face our own.

2. **Everyone has some wisdom to share.** One of the best shortcuts to any accomplishment is to find someone who has already done it and learn how she did it. The amount we can learn from even a short conversation with a

mentor is far greater than anything we can figure out on our own. Ask someone not from your culture: "What is the most important lesson you have learned?" Ask an entrepreneur or someone who has learned a new trade later in life: "How did you get started?" or "What habits have made you successful?" Learn from the both the mistakes and successes of others.

3. Ask authentic questions. Ask better questions than "How are you?" and initiate genuine conversations. "What are you working on these days?" is one of my favorites and "What concerns are weighing on you?" "What makes time stop for you?" If you are comfortable doing so, ask "What surprising thing has happened to you lately?" Sincere questions can show us new ways to see and approach life.

4. Learn from someone who will challenge you. The best learning partners are the ones who are not afraid to ask questions and challenge our assumptions. We can learn far more from the questions and ideas of people who differ from us or push us to examine our beliefs and goals.

As Muriel Rukeyser says, "The Universe is made of stories, not of atoms." Learn from every person you meet. Find out what makes them tick. Be curious about other people's goals and ideas. We can learn so much from each other's stories. There is infinite wisdom all around us. Instead of staring at your smartphone in a waiting area, take a moment to ask someone a real question face-to-face (F2F). The answer may change your life.

Questions for Reflection

- Do I know the names of my neighbors (including their kids)?
- What action might I take to create a greater sense of neighborhood where I live? (i.e., a block party, holiday gathering, or carpool).
- What country or culture do I find interesting?
- What country or culture scares me a little?
- What periods of history do I know the least about?
- Am I willing to talk with a stranger from another country to learn about them, their concerns and their history?
- What do I need to learn to grow in knowledge and empathy about cultures not my own?

Everything is related, and we human beings are united as brothers and sisters on a wonderful pilgrimage, woven together by the love God has for each creature and which also unites us in fond affection with brother sun, sister moon, brother river and mother earth. ~ Pope Francis (the 266th)

When we try to pick out anything by itself, we find it hitched to everything else in the universe. ~ John Muir

Practicing Care for Our Surroundings (Wherever We Are)

The idea that one has a share in the planet and that one can and should help care for it may seem very large and, to some, quite beyond reality. But today what happens on the other side of the world, even so far away, can affect what happens in your own home.

Cut down too many forests, foul too many rivers and seas, mess up the atmosphere and we have had it. The surface temperature can go roasting hot; the rain can turn to sulfuric acid. Sure, all living things will die but lengthening the lifecycle is possible if health and wellness are priorities.

One can ask, "Even if that were true, what could I do about it?" Well, even if one were simply to frown when people do things to mess up the planet, one would be doing something about it. Even if one only had the opinion that it was just not a good thing to wreck the planet and mentioned that opinion, one would be doing something.

Care for the planet begins in one's garden. It extends through the home, the commute to school or work, the nearby parks, roads, junkyards, forests, waste management and water-supply. Planting a tree may seem little enough but it is something.

In some countries, old people, the unemployed do not just sit around and go to pieces: they are used to care for the gardens and parks and forests, to pick up the litter and add some beauty to the world. There is no lack of resources to take care of the planet. They are mainly ignored. One notes that the Civilian Conservation Corps in the US, organized in the 1930s — no longer in existence — to absorb the energies of unemployed officers and youth, was one of the few, if not the only project of that depressed era, that created far more wealth for the state than was expended.

There are many things one can do to help take care of the planet. They begin with the idea that one should. They progress with encouragement. The planet is, after all, what we're standing on.

If others do not help safeguard and improve the environment, the way to happiness could have no roadbed to travel on at all. ~ Pope Francis

Questions for Reflection

- When do I notice my environment, what do I notice?
- What do I think about the effects of my surroundings on myself?
- When I think about actions that support the planet, what advice would I give others? Am I following my own advice?

- Who influences me the most when it comes to thinking about the importance of leaving places nicer than I've found them?
- How do people I admire behave or relate to the natural world in general?

Do Smartphones Make Us Dumb?

The smart phone isn't a perfect device, as we all know. It forces the world into a tiny screen. It runs out of battery, bandwidth, and power. It distracts us from the world around us. ~ John Battelle

We are the greatest computers in this world, but now we've created the smart phone which is smarter than us now, but we're still making dumb decisions. We have given our creations more power than we have, and that to me is dumb. ~ Bootsy Collins

On average, smartphone users spend between two to four hours every day hunched over their phones, checking email, texting, or in their apps. That's almost 1400 hours every year that people are putting their spines in a compromised position.

According to New York spine surgeon Dr. Kenneth Hansraj texting is like lifting weights but doing so unwittingly. He determined that, when you bend your head forward at 15 degrees, its weight effectively increases from 12 pounds to 27 pounds. At 45 degrees, your head exerts 49 pounds of force, and at 60 degrees, 60 pounds—this is like carrying an eight year-old child around your neck for several hours a day!images

Imagine carrying an eight year-old child around your neck for several hours a day, EVERY DAY!

"The problem is really obvious in kids" explained my own chiropractor, "stress on their neck is leading to complaints of neck pain and headaches from smartphone users, some as young as nine years old."

Why do we compulsively do what obviously hurts us?

Compulsive texting is a common disorder. In fact, 23% of teens say they send and receive over 100 messages each day. 9% say they text compulsively. That's a total of 23 out of every 100 teens saying they send and/or receive over 100 messages every day; that's a lot of messages.

Both teens and text-dependent adults are becoming even more restless, easily bored creatures and, for too many of us, our gadgets give us in abundance qualities our neurochemical systems find particularly exciting. Novelty is one.

The dopamine delivery system is activated by finding something unexpected or by the anticipation of something new. If the rewards come unpredictably — as text messages do—we get even more carried away. No wonder we called our earliest smartphones "CrackBerries."

The system is also activated by particular types of cues that a reward is coming. In order to have the maximum effect, the cues should be small, discrete, specific — like the bell Russian physiologist Ivan Pavlov rang for his dogs.

Washington State University neuroscientist Jaak Panksepp says a way to drive animals into a frenzy is to give them only tiny bits of food: This simultaneously stimulating and unsatisfying tease sends the seeking system into hyperactivity. University of Michigan professor of psychology Kent Berridge says the "ding" announcing the arrival of a text message serves as a reward cue for us. And when we respond, we get a little piece of news that makes us want more. We seek this buzz to our physical detriment.

Over time, this poor posture, or text neck, can lead to early wear and tear on our spines and eventually cause degeneration and arthritis regardless of age. Still, pain doesn't seem to register when we're getting the dopamine buzz of being "plugged in" to this random reward system.

Imagine if we keep up this bad habit what will happen to our posture, to our spines. I've been told, "The neck should have a natural reverse C-shaped curve, but patients with text neck are beginning to lose their neck's natural curve. Instead, the vertebrae in their neck are stacked on top of one another."

Without the natural curve in our spines, the joints in our neck begin to degenerate. The discs (or soft jelly-like tissue) between our vertebra eventually give out because of the pressure. This is the beginning of arthritis. With little room for nerves to exit, they become pinched and irritated. This can cause severe neck pain, stiff neck, shoulder pain and headaches.

Do you have a phone that lets you text, surf the web, and play games? That's a lot of mileage for your thumbs. Chiropractors have begun reporting cases of arthritis at the base of the thumb in younger people, possibly related to texting.

When your thumbs begin to ache, give the texting a rest. If pain continues, use your phone to make an actual call to your favorite health professional.

It's Never Too Late!

The good news? We've only been using smartphones since the 21st century, it's not too late to break these dangerous patterns. There are ways we can catch ourselves in the act of this addictive habit and switch gears. Cultivating mindfulness and choosing contrary action gives us its own neurochemical reward. We feel more confident that we are choosing what is ultimately a kinder relationship to our bodies and others,

It doesn't hurt to experiment with new behavior. Try leaving your phone at the door when you enter your dwelling. Or if going out, try leaving it in the car. Our concentration improves as a result. When we spend time with people we may feel jittery at first but this new practice can give us the capacity to be present, to listen better, to connect in more satisfying ways. But, like all habits, practice makes perfect (or good enough).

Questions for Reflection

* What's your relationship with your smartphone?
* Do you text in a daily way? Where?
* Do you have a day with no screen time?
* Are you willing to commit to making one day a week a day without social media?
* Are you able to put your phone away when you eat (alone or, *especially*, with another)?

People who say it cannot be done shouldn't interrupt those who are doing it.
~ George Bernard Shaw

Need little, want less. ~ Laozi

Build Courage

No one who amounts to anything came by it without some struggle. People born into ease — like Nepalese Prince Siddhartha — often grow restless and curious about how the "other half" live. Though it's hard to believe, a universal truism is most of us want what we don't have vs. celebrate what we do have.

The story of the Indian prince Siddhartha reveals what happens if parents spoil and shelter their children too much. He lived in opulence from birth (6th century BCE) until he ventured out around age 20 from the protective walls his parents had built for him. They wanted him to be happy and at ease and thought keeping him safe from the vagaries of life would make him sad, helpless and hopeless. They worked to protect him from any suffering.

As Siddhartha climbed outside the palace walls he came upon a very old man, a very sick man, a corpse and an ascetic. He was flabbergasted by such suffering and wondered how this could happen. Didn't everyone have his privilege?

Siddhartha sought out the wisdom of holy people — ascetics — considered infinitely wise. They told him to renounce the world, his body, all desire, and non-necessary activities. This choice would release him from all fear.

For the next six years, Siddhartha lived an ascetic life and imitated his wise mentors. Fasting, sitting without moving, inflicting bodily pain, and resisting all physical temptations seemed to leave him obsessed versus relieved from these preoccupations.

Siddhartha suddenly realized austerity was not the way to enlightenment. He then began eating, bathing and caring for himself and others in a balanced way and encouraged people to work with life instead of renouncing it. He urged others to live a full life pursuing wholeness instead of one characterized by extremism. He called this path the Middle Way.

In order to express his newfound wisdom, experientially acquired, he had to trust himself, to exercise discernment and to hold his discoveries with great respect in the face of "experts" judging him. When he was told that his new way would fail to achieve spiritual awakening. He had to resist the urge to please them.

For Siddhartha, trusting himself required wholehearted courage. According to author Brené Brown, "Courage is a heart word. The root of the word courage is *cor* which is the Latin word for heart. In one of its earliest forms, the word courage meant "To speak one's mind by telling all one's heart."

Brown's definition invites us to step up and live our experiences out loud. To speak honestly and openly about who we are and about our experiences — good and bad — requires wholeheartedness. Speaking from our hearts is what I think of as true courage. No need to slay dragons unless the dragons are critical voices or judgmental "experts" in our heads.

Questions for Reflection

- Recall a time in your life where you witnessed another act courageously.
- Remember a scene in your life when you acted courageously.
- What scares you the most (besides things like snakes, bats, spiders, etc.)?
- Who in your life would you be if you were courageous? What would you be doing the same or differently?
- If you were a superhero, what special powers would you have?

The purpose of life is not to be happy. It is to be useful, to be honorable, to be compassionate, to have it make some difference that you have lived and lived well. ~ Ralph Waldo Emerson

To seek the highest good is to live well. ~ Augustine of Hippo

Joy is Not the Absence of Pain

Some of us can feel so physically well that we believe our work is done. However, joy is not just the absence of pain; it is the gift of continued awakening. I find joy comes from ongoing and active application of the principles of wellness in my everyday life and from sharing these experiences with others.

Life presents many opportunities for deepening my insights. I need only to bring the willingness to grow and change. *The Parable of the Long Spoons* explains this idea very well and has been attributed to both Eastern and Western wisdom traditions.

One day a man said to God, "God, I would like to know what Heaven and Hell are like." God showed the man two doors. Inside the first one, in the middle of the room, was a large round table with a large pot of stew. It smelled delicious and made the man's mouth water, but the people sitting around the table were thin and sickly. They appeared to be famished. They were holding spoons with very long handles and each found it possible to reach into the pot of stew and take a spoonful, but because the handle was longer than their arms, they could not get the spoons back into their mouths.

The man shuddered at the sight of their misery and suffering. God said, "You have seen Hell."

Behind the second door, the room appeared exactly the same. There was the large round table with the large pot of wonderful stew that made the man's mouth water. The people had the same long-handled spoons, but they were well nourished and plump, laughing and talking.

The man said, "I don't understand."

God smiled. "It is simple," he said, "Love only requires one skill. These people learned early on to share and feed one another. While the greedy only think of themselves."

Sometimes, thinking of our personal gratification, we tend to forget our interdependence with everyone and everything around us. As the parable makes clear, not to help our fellow human beings simply means harming our very selves, since we are all connected on the deepest level.

Questions for Reflection
- Can I honestly say, "I am joyful?"
- When I was a child, what did I consider important?
- How has my sense of happiness changed over the last ten years?
- Do I feel a sense of generosity in my everyday life?

- Have I extended any form of help to my fellows? What has that looked like in the past? What might it look like in my future?
- Is there anything I'm too afraid to do to outgrow?
- Is it okay to be who I am today?

I have done my best. That is about all the philosophy of living one needs.
~ Lin Yutang

Life is not to live merely, but to live well. ~ Eric Lubbock

Cultivating A Framework for Living

One of my favorite stories about life is told by a Buddhist Abbess, Pema Chodron. Wholehearted living is described as a man clinging to a rope on a steep hillside. A fresh strawberry tenuously dangling on a branch is almost out of reach. The tale is called "Tigers above, tigers below." According to Pema, we all dangle on the hill of life with the pacing tigers of death and birth reminding us of our impermanence. This lone and very ripe strawberry called wholehearted living awaits our savoring. Do we have the courage to reach out and pluck it? "This is actually the predicament that we are always in, in terms of our birth and death. Each moment is just what it is. It might be the only moment of our life; it might be the only strawberry we'll ever eat. We could get depressed about it, or we could finally appreciate it and delight in the preciousness of every single moment of our life."

By reading the brief essays in this book, by now, you know what I believe leads to wholehearted living. Each one of these principles laid out before you make up what I believe supports our wholehearted health and wellness. I have seen many of my own clients grow exponentially in feeling more flexible and peaceful when they practice even one of these suggestions above.

But, dear reader, I recommend you find out for yourself what supports your own health and wellbeing. Hopefully you have been taking the opportunities within each essay to reflect and question your own habits of thinking and acting. Finding what speaks to you is what matters. What doesn't inspire you in this book can be easily left behind; one thing is for sure, what I think is how I live (for good or for ill).

By becoming aware of our fearful thoughts and positive and habits, we will continue to build (and build on) our healthy foundation for courageous living. And as you must know by now *to live wholeheartedly is to live well.*

Questions for Reflection

- Of all the questions in this book, which one has helped you the most?
- Where have you disagreed with an idea or belief stated in this book?
- Who do you know that could be helped by the ideas within this book?
- What new idea will you put into practice for your own health and wellbeing?
- What would you add to the mix of ideas we have shared with you in these essays?
- Are you willing to write and let me know what you would add and what you thought about this work? I want to hear from you and can be reached at info@EmboldenU.com

21 Ways to Consider What Matters Most by James Hollis

1. THE CHOICE IS YOURS:
Realize that your life is something you choose every day, whether you are paying attention or not. And that it is now time to pay attention.

2. TIME TO GROW UP:
Grow Up. Growing up means that we truly take responsibility for our lives, for how they are turning out, and stop expecting others to make those decisions for us.

3. LET GO OF THE OLD:
Pay attention to how much of your daily behavior is in service to old anxiety management systems that, once necessary, now bind you to a disempowering past.

4. RECOVER PERSONAL AUTHORITY:
Recover personal authority: what is true for you, really, and now find the courage to live that truth.

5. SEEK TO MAKE AMENDS:
Ask others where you have injured them, where they see you limiting yourself, and vow to change those behaviors.

6. STEP OUT FROM UNDER THE PARENTAL SHADE:
Consider where you are still carrying, or compensating for, the un-lived life of your Mother, the un-lived life of your Father.

7. VOW TO GET UNSTUCK:
Reflect on where you are stuck, and what old fear is keeping you stuck.

8. COME BACK TO YOUR TASK: Identify what task you need to address, the flight from which will diminish your life.

9. CHOOSE THE PATH OF ENLARGEMENT:
Ask of any important life choice: does this path enlarge me or diminish me — and act on your conclusion.

10. WHAT GIFT HAVE YOU BEEN WITHHOLDING FROM THE WORLD:
What wishes to come into the world through you, and only your fears keep you from serving it?

11. SEE THE OLD SELF-DESTRUCTIVE PATTERNS:
Notice the patterns which keep showing up in your intimate relationships, and from whence do they arise in your history?

12. WHAT IS THE BIGGER PICTURE FOR YOU?
Where do you stand in relationship to what is larger than you, that which asks more of you?

13. CHOOSE MEANING OVER HAPPINESS:
A life of happiness is transient; the search for meaning is life-long.

14. HONOR, FINALLY, WHAT YOU LEFT BEHIND:
What parts of yourself did you leave behind, perhaps necessarily then, but which cry out for your recovery of them, for your honoring of them?

15. EXORCISE THE GHOSTS OF THE PAST WHICH BIND YOU:
What old guilt or shame inhibits you today, and how can you grow larger than their inhibiting powers?

16. FREE YOUR CHILDREN FROM YOU:
Free your children from your own un-lived life, your expectations that they ratify your values, and release them as you wished released from the expectations of your parents.

17. BESTOW LOVE ON THE UNLOVEABLE PARTS OF YOU:
Accept that fact that we all are flawed, which does not mean that we are not worthy of love, of respect, and of the power to redo our lives.

18. HONOR THE DIFFERENCE BETWEEN DUTY AND CALLING:
Know the difference between work and vocation, that one is a duty and one is a calling, and that in the end, a calling is more important than anything.

19. EXPLORE WHAT ONCE MOVED YOU MOST:
What fired your imagination in the past, aroused your curiosity and passion? Those energies are still there, waiting for release and affirmation.

20. SIEZE PERMISSION TO BE WHO YOU REALLY ARE:
Where are you still looking for permission to live your life, and who do you think will give it to you today?

21. LIVE THE EXAMINED LIFE:
Keep asking yourself, "What matters most?" lest you be living someone else's life, or simply staying on automatic pilot.

Questions for Reflection

- What have you learned from reading this list?
- What would you add or remove?
- How can I support you in well-rounded wellness? Please let me know by reaching out to me through my website: EmboldenU.com

Life is not so much about beginnings and endings as it is about going on and on and on. It is about muddling through the middle. ~ Anna Quindlen

It has been a pleasure, dear reader, to join you in finding **ways** to wholehearted wellness. Notice I did not say THE way; that would be arrogant. No one culture, no one person has all the answers no matter how hard they may try to convince others and themselves. I have come to find that there are multiple ways to finding wellness.

Wholehearted wellness works like a wagon wheel with many spokes, each one must be balanced to roll smoothly. The road can be bumpy and the destination ephemeral. The journey requires full attention. Though we are all responsible to attend to our own body, mind and spirit, we trudge the long road together — friend and stranger — and help each other all along the way.

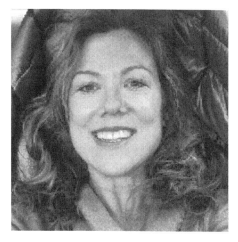

Dr. Jennifer Manlowe has been involved in wholehearted wellness for decades. Since 1993, she has been an author many times over and given lectures and workshops throughout the United States, Europe, Canada, Central America, the Caribbean, Russia and China. She has appeared as a guest on several radio shows and has been featured in many online magazines around the world.

She is the founder of _Embolden U: Share Your Gifts with the World!_ a successful international consulting practice with creative clarity programs and courses designed to give people the tools to understand and express who they are and what they want to create in their wholehearted life.

NOTES:

NOTES:

Made in the USA
San Bernardino, CA
19 March 2017